The Real Truth About Aging and Longevity

TABLE OF CONTENTS

<u>Part 1: Demystifying Aging</u>

1. **The Biology of Time:**

   The scientific understanding of aging at the cellular and molecular level, examining key theories like telomere shortening, DNA damage, and epigenetic changes.

2. **Beyond Genes: The Environmental Symphony:**

   The myth of aging as solely genetic, outlining the significant role of environmental factors like diet, exercise, stress, and pollution.

3. **Lifespan vs. Healthspan: Redefining the Goal:**

   Shift the focus from simply lengthening lifespan to optimizing health span, emphasizing the importance of quality of life in later years.

4. **Evolutionary Trade-offs: Why We Age:**

   The evolutionary perspective on aging, explaining why natural selection doesn't favor indefinite lifespan and exploring the potential benefits of aging mechanisms.

5. **Myths and Misconceptions about Aging:**

   Common myths and misinformation surrounding aging, including anti-aging miracle cures, fountain-of-youth legends, and age-related stereotyp

<u>Part 2: The Blueprint for Longevity</u>

6. **Diet: Fueling the Aging Engine:**

The crucial role of nutrition in promoting longevity, discussing optimal dietary patterns, essential nutrients, and the impact of food choices on cellular health.

7. **Exercise: Moving Towards Vitality**

The science behind exercise's anti-aging effects, outlining effective exercise routines, and addressing age-related limitations and adaptations.

8. **Sleep: Restoring Rejuvenation:**

the importance of quality sleep for cellular repair and cognitive function, providing tips for improving sleep hygiene and addressing sleep disturbances in older adults.

9. **Stress Management: Calming the Clock:**

The negative impacts of chronic stress on aging and longevity, offering practical strategies for stress reduction, relaxation techniques, and building resilience.

10. **Mental Engagement: Keeping the Mind Sharp:**

The link between mental activity and cognitive health in aging, outlining brain-training exercises, lifelong learning, and fostering social connections.

Part 3: The Future of Aging

11. **Emerging Technologies: The Longevity Toolbox:**

The cutting-edge advancements in biotechnology, gene editing, and personalized medicine with potential to positively impact aging and extend lifespan.

## 12.	The Ethics of Longevity: Living Longer, Living Better:

Ethical considerations surrounding longevity research and interventions, exploring issues of resource allocation, equity, and potential societal implications.

## 13.	Rethinking Aging: A Paradigm Shift:

Advocate for a cultural shift in perceptions of aging, promoting active, engaged, and meaningful elderhood as a valuable stage of life.

## 14.	Individual Action, Collective Impact:

Empower readers to take personal responsibility for their own health and longevity, while advocating for public policy changes and scientific research advancements.

15. Living with Purpose:

Embracing the Aging Journey

INTRODUCTION

The concept of aging refers to the natural and progressive process of changes that occur in living organisms as they grow older over time. It is a universal phenomenon that affects all living beings, from single-celled organisms to complex multicellular organisms like humans. Aging is a fundamental aspect of the life cycle and is characterized by a gradual decline in physiological and functional abilities, leading to increased vulnerability to age-related diseases and ultimately death.

Aging is a complex and multifaceted process, influenced by a combination of genetic, cellular, and environmental factors. While the aging process is a natural part of life, its exact mechanisms and underlying causes are still subjects of ongoing research and investigation.

Key aspects of the concept of aging include:

1.Biological Changes: Aging involves a wide range of biological changes that occur at various levels of organization, from the cellular level to tissues, organs, and systems. These changes can include alterations in cellular metabolism, DNA damage, impaired protein synthesis, and decreased cellular repair mechanisms.

2.Cellular Senescence: One of the crucial aspects of aging is cellular senescence, where cells lose their ability to divide and replicate effectively. This contributes to a decline in tissue and organ function over time.

3.Telomere Shortening: Telomeres, protective caps at the ends of chromosomes, shorten with each cell division. As telomeres shorten, cell division becomes less efficient, leading to cellular aging and eventually cell death.

4.Accumulation of Damage: Over time, cells and tissues accumulate damage from various sources, including exposure to environmental toxins, radiation, and metabolic byproducts. This damage can lead to a decline in overall organ function and contribute to the aging process.

5.Genetic and Epigenetic Influences: Genetic factors play a significant role in determining an organism's potential lifespan and susceptibility to age-related diseases. Epigenetic modifications, which alter gene expression without changing the underlying

DNA sequence, also influence how genes behave during the aging process.

6.Environmental Factors: Lifestyle choices, diet, exercise, exposure to pollutants, and other environmental factors can accelerate or decelerate the aging process. A healthy lifestyle can promote healthy aging and delay the onset of age-related diseases.

7.Longevity and Aging Research: Scientists and researchers are continuously studying aging to better understand its mechanisms and find ways to promote healthy aging and extend human lifespan.

It's essential to note that aging is a dynamic and complex process, and individuals may experience it differently based on their genetic makeup, lifestyle choices, and environmental factors. While aging brings about physical and cognitive changes, it also presents opportunities for personal growth, wisdom, and meaningful experiences.

Understanding aging is crucial for addressing the challenges and opportunities associated with an aging population and promoting well-being and quality of life for people of all ages.

As our understanding of aging continues to evolve, so does our ability to develop interventions and strategies to support healthy aging and improve overall longevity.

DEDICATION

To all those who embrace the beauty of aging with resilience, grace, and an unwavering spirit. May this exploration into the profound journey of life's later chapters serve as a guide, a source of inspiration, and a celebration of the richness that comes with every passing year. Here's to a world where every individual is empowered to live with purpose, finding meaning in each moment and embracing the aging journey with hope, optimism, and a heart full of gratitude.

DR. PAUL BELL

Part one

Demystifying Aging

CHAPTER ONE

THE BIOLOGY OF TIME

The biology of time, particularly in the context of aging, is a fascinating and complex area of study that involves various cellular and molecular processes. Scientists have been exploring the mechanisms underlying aging to gain insights into the factors that contribute to the gradual decline in biological functions over time. Here are some key aspects of the biology of time and aging:

Telomere Shortening:

Telomeres are protective caps at the ends of chromosomes, consisting of repetitive DNA sequences.

With each cell division, telomeres gradually shorten, and when they become critically short, cells may enter a state of senescence or undergo apoptosis (cell death).

This process is often associated with the Hayflick limit, which describes the finite number of divisions a cell can undergo.

DNA Damage:

Over time, DNA can experience various forms of damage due to environmental factors, radiation, toxins, and normal metabolic processes.

Accumulated DNA damage can lead to mutations and genomic instability, contributing to aging and age-related diseases.

Cells have mechanisms like DNA repair processes to fix damage, but their efficiency can decline with age.

Epigenetic Changes:

Epigenetics involves modifications to DNA and associated proteins that regulate gene expression without altering the underlying DNA sequence.

Changes in DNA methylation, histone modification, and non-coding RNA profiles can influence gene activity.

Epigenetic alterations play a role in aging and age-related diseases, affecting cellular function and contributing to the aging process.

Mitochondrial Dysfunction:

Mitochondria are cellular organelles responsible for energy production through oxidative phosphorylation.

Over time, mitochondria can experience damage, leading to decreased energy production and increased generation of reactive oxygen species (ROS).

Mitochondrial dysfunction is implicated in aging, as it contributes to cellular decline and the progression of age-related diseases.

Cellular Senescence:

Cellular senescence is a state in which cells cease to divide and undergo functional changes.

Senescent cells can accumulate over time, contributing to tissue dysfunction and inflammation.

Senescence is linked to various age-related conditions, and strategies to remove or rejuvenate senescent cells are being explored as potential interventions for aging.

Understanding the biology of time and aging at the cellular and molecular levels provides a foundation for developing potential interventions to slow down or reverse the aging process. Ongoing research aims to unravel the intricate mechanisms involved and identify strategies for promoting healthy aging and extending lifespan.

CHAPTER TWO

BEYOND GENES: THE ENVIRONMENTAL SYMPHONY

De-bunk the myth of aging as solely genetic, outlining the significant role of environmental factors like diet, exercise, stress, and pollution.

While genetics plays a crucial role in aging, it is increasingly clear that environmental factors have a profound impact on the aging process. The interaction between genes and the environment, known as epigenetics, emphasizes that lifestyle and external influences can significantly influence how genes are expressed. Here are some key environmental factors that contribute to the aging process:

Diet:

Nutrition is a critical determinant of health and aging. A balanced and nutritious diet provides essential nutrients that support cellular functions and repair mechanisms.

Caloric restriction and intermittent fasting have been linked to longevity and improved health outcomes, influencing metabolic pathways and cellular stress responses.

Exercise:

Regular physical activity is associated with numerous health benefits, including improved cardiovascular health, enhanced metabolism, and maintenance of muscle mass.

Exercise also influences gene expression and cellular processes, contributing to overall well-being and potentially slowing down the aging process.

Stress:

Chronic stress can have detrimental effects on health and accelerate the aging process. It triggers the release of stress hormones, such as cortisol, which, when chronically elevated, can contribute to inflammation and cellular damage.

Stress management strategies, such as mindfulness and relaxation techniques, may mitigate the negative impact of stress on aging.

Pollution and Environmental Toxins:

Exposure to environmental pollutants, such as air and water contaminants, heavy metals, and pesticides, can contribute to oxidative stress and inflammation.

Long-term exposure to these pollutants may accelerate aging and increase the risk of age-related diseases.

Social and Psychological Factors:

Social connections, mental health, and lifestyle choices also play a crucial role in aging. Loneliness and social isolation have been associated with negative health outcomes, while positive social interactions can contribute to overall well-being.

Cognitive stimulation and a mentally active lifestyle may help maintain cognitive function as individual's age.

Sleep:

Quality sleep is essential for cellular repair, cognitive function, and overall health. Sleep deprivation and disturbances in sleep patterns can contribute to accelerated aging and increase the risk of chronic diseases.

UV Radiation:

Exposure to ultraviolet (UV) radiation from the sun can lead to skin aging and increase the risk of skin cancers. Protecting the skin through the use of sunscreen and other preventive measures can slow down the aging effects of UV radiation.

Debunking the myth of aging as solely genetic highlights the importance of lifestyle choices and environmental factors in shaping the aging process. While genetics provides the blueprint, the environment can modulate gene expression and influence the trajectory of aging. Adopting a healthy lifestyle, including a balanced diet, regular exercise, stress management, and minimizing exposure to environmental toxins, can contribute to healthy aging and improve overall well-being.

CHAPTER THREE

LIFESPAN VS. HEALTHSPAN

Redefining the Goal: Shift the focus from simply lengthening lifespan to optimizing healthspan, emphasizing the importance of quality of life in later years

The traditional focus on increasing lifespan has been a significant goal in medical and scientific communities. However, there is a growing recognition that mere extension of life does not necessarily equate to improved well-being. Shifting the emphasis from lifespan to healthspan represents a redefinition of the ultimate goal, highlighting the importance of optimizing the quality of life during the aging process. Here are key points in understanding and promoting healthspan:

Lifespan vs. Healthspan:

Lifespan: The total number of years a person lives.

Healthspan: The number of years an individual lives in good health, without significant disease or disability.

Quality of Life:

Focusing on healthspan emphasizes the importance of maintaining physical and mental well-being throughout the entire lifespan.

The goal is not just to extend life but to ensure that those additional years are characterized by vitality, functionality, and a high quality of life.

Prevention and Early Intervention:

Emphasizing healthspan involves a shift towards preventive healthcare and early intervention strategies.

Identifying and addressing risk factors for age-related diseases early on can contribute to better health outcomes and an extended period of healthy living.

Lifestyle Factors:

Healthy lifestyle choices, including a balanced diet, regular physical activity, and stress management, play a crucial role in optimizing healthspan.

Addressing modifiable risk factors can help prevent or delay the onset of chronic diseases associated with aging.

Cognitive Health:

Maintaining cognitive function is a key component of healthspan. Strategies that support brain health, such as cognitive stimulation, social engagement, and a healthy diet, are important for optimizing overall well-being.

Functional Independence:

Healthspan is not just about living longer but living independently and with a high degree of functional capability.

Maintaining mobility, muscle strength, and sensory functions contributes to a more active and fulfilling lifestyle in later years.

Social and Emotional Well-being:

Social connections, emotional resilience, and a positive outlook on life are integral to health span.

Strategies that promote mental and emotional well-being, such as social engagement and stress reduction, contribute to a healthier and more satisfying life.

Personalized Approaches:

Recognizing the diversity in individual health trajectories calls for personalized approaches to healthcare and interventions.

Tailoring strategies based on genetic predispositions, lifestyle factors, and individual health profiles can optimize outcomes for each person.

By shifting the focus from merely increasing lifespan to optimizing healthspan, the goal becomes not only to add years to life but to add life to years. This paradigm shift encourages a holistic approach to aging that prioritizes the maintenance of physical, mental, and emotional well-being. Ultimately, the aim is to enable individuals to lead longer, healthier, and more fulfilling lives.

CHAPTER FOUR

EVOLUTIONARY TRADE-OFFS: WHY WE AGE

In this chapter, we shall endeavor to go into the evolutionary perspective on aging, explaining why natural selection doesn't favor indefinite lifespan and exploring the potential benefits of aging mechanisms.

The evolutionary perspective on aging provides insights into why organisms, including humans, experience aging despite the apparent disadvantage of reduced fitness and mortality. Several theories attempt to explain the evolutionary trade-offs and the reasons why natural selection doesn't favor indefinite lifespan. Here are some key aspects of the evolutionary perspective on aging:

Antagonistic Pleiotropy:

The antagonistic pleiotropy hypothesis suggests that certain genes that have positive effects early in life may have negative effects later in life.

Evolutionary pressures may favor genes that enhance reproductive success and survival during the reproductive years, even if those same genes contribute to aging and decreased fitness in later life.

Disposable Soma Theory:

The disposable soma theory proposes that resources allocated to reproduction are prioritized over those invested in somatic maintenance and repair.

Evolution may favor allocating resources for successful reproduction, even if it results in the gradual deterioration of the body over time.

Mutation Accumulation:

The mutation accumulation theory suggests that harmful mutations with late-life effects can accumulate in a population because natural selection is less effective at eliminating them in older individuals.

Mutations that impact health and survival later in life may not be strongly selected against, as they have minimal impact on reproductive success.

Evolutionary Senescence:

Evolutionary senescence refers to the decline in fitness with age, and it is thought to result from a combination of genetic, cellular, and environmental factors.

Over time, selective pressures decrease as individuals age, allowing deleterious mutations to accumulate and influence the aging process.

Evolutionary Benefits of Aging Mechanisms:

Aging mechanisms, such as programmed cell death (apoptosis) and cellular senescence, may serve beneficial roles in specific contexts.

Apoptosis can eliminate damaged or malfunctioning cells, preventing the spread of harmful mutations.

Cellular senescence may contribute to tissue repair and wound healing, as well as play a role in preventing the development of cancer by halting the division of potentially harmful cells.

Group Selection and Altruistic Aging:

Some theories propose that there may be benefits to the group or community that come from having older individuals with accumulated knowledge and experience.

Altruistic behaviors, where older individuals invest resources in the well-being of their offspring or the group, could confer advantages to the group as a whole.

Evolutionary Adaptations to Specific Environments:

The pace of aging and lifespan can vary across species and populations based on their specific ecological and environmental contexts.

Evolution may shape aging patterns in response to specific challenges and opportunities present in particular environments.

While aging may seem counterintuitive from an individual fitness perspective, understanding the evolutionary trade-offs provides a more nuanced view of the complexities involved. Aging mechanisms may have evolved as compromises that optimize reproductive success and survival in specific ecological and social contexts. Additionally, the potential benefits of aging mechanisms, such as apoptosis and cellular senescence, highlight their adaptive roles in maintaining overall organismal health.

CHAPTER FIVE

MYTHS AND MISCONCEPTIONS ABOUT AGING

Common myths and misinformation surrounding aging, including anti-aging miracle cures, fountain-of-youth legends, and age-related stereotypes

There are numerous myths and misconceptions about aging that persist in society, often fueled by misinformation, cultural beliefs, and a desire for quick fixes. It's important to dispel these myths to promote a more accurate understanding of the aging process. Here are some common myths and misconceptions about aging:

Myth: Aging Is Inevitably Associated with Poor Health:

Fact: While aging is a natural process, not everyone experiences poor health in old age. Healthy lifestyle choices, including a balanced diet, regular exercise, and stress management, can contribute to maintaining good health throughout life.

Myth: Anti-Aging Products Can Reverse the Aging Process:

Fact: Many products claim to have anti-aging properties, but there is no scientifically proven method to reverse the aging process. Skincare products can help with skin health, but they cannot fundamentally change the biological aging of the entire body.

Myth: Aging Only Affects the Elderly:

Fact: Aging is a lifelong process that begins at conception. Biological, cognitive, and social changes occur at different stages of life, and the effects of aging are cumulative. It's not limited to the elderly population.

Myth: Aging Equals Memory Decline:

Fact: While cognitive decline can occur with age, not everyone experiences severe memory problems. Healthy lifestyle choices, mental stimulation, and social engagement can support cognitive function in old age.

Myth: Older People Are Technologically Inept:

Fact: Many older individuals are proficient with technology, and there's a wide range of technological literacy among people of all ages. Older adults can and do adapt to new technologies.

Myth: Aging Means Loss of Interest in Sex:

Fact: Sexual desire and activity can continue into old age. While there may be physiological changes, maintaining a healthy sex life is possible with communication, emotional intimacy, and adaptability.

Myth: Older Adults Are Unable to Learn New Things:

Fact: Lifelong learning is possible at any age. Older adults can acquire new skills, pursue education, and engage in intellectually stimulating activities that promote cognitive health.

Myth: Older People Are Lonely and Unhappy:

Fact: Social isolation and loneliness can affect individuals at any age. However, many older adults maintain active social lives, engage in meaningful relationships, and report high levels of life satisfaction.

Myth: Aging Is a Uniform Process for Everyone:

Fact: Aging is highly individualized, influenced by genetics, lifestyle, and environmental factors. People age at different rates, and the impact of aging varies widely among individuals.

Myth: Older Workers Are Less Productive:

Fact: Older workers can be highly productive, experienced, and valuable contributors to the workforce. Age does not necessarily correlate with decreased productivity or competence.

Dispelling these myths helps combat age-related stereotypes, promotes a more positive view of aging, and encourages a realistic and informed perspective on the aging process. It's essential to recognize the diversity and resilience of older individuals and challenge unfounded beliefs that can contribute to ageism and discrimination.

Part 2:

The Blueprint for Longevity

CHAPTER SIX

DIET: FUELING THE AGING ENGINE

We shall Explore the crucial role of nutrition in promoting longevity, discussing optimal dietary patterns, essential nutrients, and the impact of food choices on cellular health in this chapter.

Diet plays a crucial role in promoting longevity and overall health throughout the aging process. Proper nutrition provides essential nutrients that support cellular function, protect against oxidative stress, and contribute to the maintenance of various bodily functions. Here are key aspects of the role of diet in fueling the aging engine:

Balanced Diet:

A balanced diet includes a variety of foods from all food groups, providing a mix of macronutrients (carbohydrates, proteins, and fats) and micronutrients (vitamins and minerals).

Emphasizing a diverse range of nutrient-dense foods supports overall health and helps prevent nutritional deficiencies.

Caloric Restriction and Intermittent Fasting:

Caloric restriction, without malnutrition, has been associated with increased lifespan and healthspan in various animal studies.

Intermittent fasting, which involves cycles of eating and fasting, may also have health benefits, including improved metabolic health and cellular repair.

Antioxidant-Rich Foods:

Antioxidants help combat oxidative stress, a process associated with aging and age-related diseases. Fruits and vegetables, particularly those rich in vitamins C and E, beta-carotene, and other antioxidants, contribute to cellular health.

Omega-3 Fatty Acids:

Omega-3 fatty acids, found in fatty fish (such as salmon and mackerel), flaxseeds, and walnuts, have anti-inflammatory properties and support cardiovascular and brain health.

Protein Intake:

Adequate protein intake is essential for maintaining muscle mass, which tends to decline with age. Including sources of lean protein, such as poultry, fish, beans, and dairy, supports muscle health and overall bodily functions.

Fiber-Rich Foods:

Dietary fiber, found in whole grains, fruits, vegetables, and legumes, supports digestive health and helps regulate blood sugar levels and cholesterol.

Hydration:

Staying adequately hydrated is crucial for overall health, especially as dehydration can be more common in older adults. Water supports digestion, nutrient absorption, and temperature regulation.

Calcium and Vitamin D

Calcium and vitamin D are important for bone health. Dairy products, leafy greens, and fortified foods contribute to calcium intake, while vitamin D is synthesized by the skin in response to sunlight.

Minimizing Processed Foods and Added Sugars:

Limiting the intake of processed foods, sugary beverages, and added sugars is essential for maintaining metabolic health and preventing conditions such as obesity and type 2 diabetes.

Individualized Nutrition:

Nutrition needs can vary among individuals based on factors such as age, gender, activity level, and health status.

Consulting with a healthcare professional or registered dietitian can help tailor dietary recommendations to individual needs.

Mindful Eating:

Paying attention to hunger and fullness cues, practicing mindful eating, and enjoying meals in a relaxed environment can contribute to a healthier relationship with food and support overall well-being.

Adopting a nutrient-rich, balanced diet that meets individual needs is a cornerstone of healthy aging. It provides the necessary building blocks for cellular repair, supports immune function, and helps prevent age-related diseases. Combined with other healthy lifestyle choices, such as regular physical activity and stress management, a nutritious diet contributes to promoting longevity and optimizing the quality of life in later years.

CHAPTER SEVEN

EXERCISE: MOVING TOWARDS VITALITY

Examine the science behind exercise's anti-aging effects, outlining effective exercise routines, and addressing age-related limitations and adaptations.

Exercise is a powerful tool in promoting vitality and mitigating the effects of aging. The science behind exercise's anti-aging effects is grounded in its impact on various physiological processes, from cellular function to overall health. Here's an exploration of the anti-aging effects of exercise, effective exercise routines, and considerations for age-related limitations and adaptations:

Cellular Health:

Exercise has been shown to have positive effects on cellular health, including mitigating oxidative stress and inflammation.

Regular physical activity supports mitochondrial function and cellular repair processes, contributing to overall cellular resilience.

Cardiovascular Health:

Aerobic exercise, such as walking, jogging, and cycling, improves cardiovascular health by enhancing heart and lung function, reducing the risk of cardiovascular diseases, and improving circulation.

Strength Training and Muscle Mass:

Resistance or strength training helps maintain and build muscle mass, which tends to decline with age.

Preserving muscle mass is crucial for maintaining functional independence, preventing falls, and supporting metabolic health.

Bone Density:

Weight-bearing exercises, including walking, running, and resistance training, stimulate bone formation and help maintain bone density, reducing the risk of osteoporosis and fractures.

Neurological Benefits:

Exercise has positive effects on cognitive function and may reduce the risk of age-related cognitive decline and neurodegenerative diseases.

Both aerobic exercise and activities that challenge balance and coordination contribute to brain health.

Hormonal Regulation:

Exercise influences the release of hormones, including endorphins that improve mood, and growth factors that support tissue repair and maintenance.

Flexibility and Mobility:

Activities that enhance flexibility and mobility, such as stretching and yoga, contribute to joint health and help maintain a full range of motion.

Effective Exercise Routines:

A well-rounded exercise routine should include a mix of aerobic exercises, strength training, flexibility exercises, and balance and coordination activities.

Aim for at least 150 minutes of moderate-intensity aerobic exercise per week and include strength training exercises at least twice a week.

Considerations for Age-Related Limitations:

Individuals should tailor their exercise routines to accommodate any existing health conditions or physical limitations.

Low-impact activities, such as swimming or cycling, can be beneficial for those with joint issues.

Consulting with a healthcare professional or fitness expert can help design a personalized exercise plan.

Adaptations with Age:

As individuals age, it may be necessary to modify exercise routines to accommodate changes in flexibility, balance, and muscle mass.

Incorporating exercises that focus on stability, coordination, and flexibility becomes increasingly important.

Consistency is Key:

Long-term, consistent exercise is crucial for reaping the full anti-aging benefits.

Finding enjoyable activities and incorporating them into a regular routine helps maintain motivation and adherence.

It's important to note that the benefits of exercise extend beyond physical health; they also contribute to mental and emotional well-being. As with any lifestyle change, it's advisable to consult with healthcare professionals, especially for those with pre-existing health conditions. By adopting a comprehensive and tailored exercise routine, individuals can promote vitality, enhance overall health, and better navigate the aging process.

CHAPTER EIGHT

SLEEP: RESTORING REJUVENATION

Quality sleep is a crucial component of overall health and well-being, playing a vital role in cellular repair, cognitive function, and various physiological processes. Understanding the importance of sleep and adopting good sleep hygiene practices is particularly relevant for promoting rejuvenation, especially in older adults. Here's an exploration of the significance of sleep, tips for improving sleep hygiene, and considerations for addressing sleep disturbances in older individuals:

Cellular Repair and Growth Hormone Release:

During deep sleep, the body undergoes important processes of cellular repair and growth hormone release, contributing to physical restoration and overall well-being.

Cognitive Function and Memory Consolidation:

Sleep is essential for cognitive function, memory consolidation, and learning. Adequate and quality sleep supports optimal brain function and helps maintain cognitive performance.

Emotional Well-being:

Sleep plays a crucial role in emotional regulation and resilience. Lack of sleep can contribute to mood disturbances, irritability, and an increased risk of mental health issues.

Immune Function:

Quality sleep is linked to a robust immune system. Adequate rest supports the body's ability to defend against infections and illnesses.

Hormonal Balance:

Sleep influences the balance of hormones, including those that regulate hunger and satiety. Poor sleep can contribute to disruptions in appetite regulation and potentially lead to weight gain.

Tips for Improving Sleep Hygiene:

Consistent Sleep Schedule: Going to bed and waking up at the same time every day helps regulate the body's internal clock.

Create a Relaxing Bedtime Routine: Engage in calming activities before bedtime, such as reading, gentle stretching, or meditation, to signal to the body that it's time to wind down.

Comfortable Sleep Environment: Ensure the bedroom is conducive to sleep by maintaining a comfortable temperature, minimizing noise and light, and investing in a comfortable mattress and pillows.

Limit Screen Time: Reduce exposure to screens, including phones, tablets, and computers, at least an hour before bedtime, as the blue light emitted can interfere with the production of the sleep hormone melatonin.

Watch Diet and Caffeine Intake: Avoid heavy meals and caffeine close to bedtime, as they can disrupt sleep.

Addressing Sleep Disturbances in Older Adults:

Understand Changes in Sleep Patterns: Older adults may experience changes in sleep architecture, including lighter sleep, more frequent awakenings, and a tendency to go to bed and wake up earlier.

Regular Physical Activity: Engaging in regular physical activity, preferably earlier in the day, can promote better sleep in older adults.

Limit Naps: While short naps can be beneficial, long or irregular napping during the day may interfere with nighttime sleep.

Manage Medication Effects: Some medications may affect sleep. Consult with a healthcare professional to review medications and discuss potential adjustments.

Consulting Healthcare Professionals:

Persistent sleep disturbances or conditions such as insomnia may require consultation with healthcare professionals, including sleep specialists or primary care physicians, for a comprehensive assessment and guidance.

Recognizing the importance of quality sleep and adopting effective sleep hygiene practices contributes to overall health and vitality, particularly in older adults. Making sleep a priority and addressing sleep-related issues can enhance the quality of life and support healthy aging.

CHAPTER NINE

STRESS MANAGEMENT: CALMING THE CLOCK

Explore the negative impacts of chronic stress on aging and longevity, offering practical strategies for stress reduction, relaxation techniques, and building resilience.

Chronic stress can have profound negative impacts on aging and longevity, affecting both physical and mental well-being. Understanding the relationship between stress and aging and adopting effective stress management strategies are essential for promoting overall health and resilience. Here's an exploration of the negative impacts of chronic stress, practical strategies for stress reduction, relaxation techniques, and building resilience:

Negative Impacts of Chronic Stress on Aging:

Chronic stress is associated with increased inflammation, which plays a role in various age-related diseases, including cardiovascular disease, diabetes, and neurodegenerative disorders.

Stress can accelerate cellular aging by affecting telomere length, contributing to premature aging at the cellular level.

Mental health issues such as anxiety and depression, often linked to chronic stress, can impact cognitive function and quality of life in older adults.

Practical Strategies for Stress Reduction:

Mindfulness and Meditation: Practices such as mindfulness meditation can help manage stress by promoting relaxation and cultivating awareness of the present moment.

Deep Breathing Exercises: Deep, slow breathing can activate the body's relaxation response, reducing stress hormones and promoting a sense of calm.

Regular Exercise: Physical activity is a powerful stress reliever, promoting the release of endorphins and enhancing mood. Activities such as walking, yoga, and tai chi can be particularly beneficial.

Time Management: Organizing tasks and setting realistic goals can help reduce feelings of overwhelm and stress.

Social Support: Maintaining strong social connections and seeking support from friends, family, or support groups can provide a valuable buffer against stress.

Hobbies and Leisure Activities: Engaging in activities that bring joy and relaxation, such as reading, gardening, or listening to music, can be effective stress management tools.

Relaxation Techniques:

Progressive Muscle Relaxation (PMR): Involves tensing and then relaxing different muscle groups to release physical tension.

Guided Imagery: Involves visualizing calming and peaceful scenes to promote relaxation and reduce stress.

Biofeedback: Utilizes electronic monitoring to provide real-time information about physiological processes, helping individuals learn to control bodily functions and reduce stress.

Building Resilience:

Cognitive Restructuring: Developing a positive and adaptive mindset by challenging and changing negative thought patterns.

Mindfulness-Based Stress Reduction (MBSR): Programs that incorporate mindfulness meditation and awareness techniques to enhance resilience and cope with stress.

Emotional Intelligence: Developing the ability to recognize and manage one's emotions and navigate interpersonal relationships effectively.

Adaptive Coping Strategies: Encouraging problem-solving and seeking solutions to stressors rather than dwelling on negative emotions.

Healthy Lifestyle Habits:

Balanced Diet: Nutrient-rich foods support overall health, and certain nutrients can positively impact mood and stress resilience.

Adequate Sleep: Prioritize good sleep hygiene to support physical and mental well-being.

Regular Physical Activity: Exercise not only helps relieve stress but also contributes to overall resilience and well-being.

Seeking Professional Support:

If stress becomes overwhelming or chronic, seeking guidance from mental health professionals, such as therapists or counselors, can provide effective coping strategies.

Adopting stress management strategies and building resilience is crucial for mitigating the negative impacts of chronic stress on aging. By incorporating these practices into daily life, individuals can promote overall well-being, enhance longevity, and navigate the aging process with greater resilience and vitality.

Part 3:

The Future of Aging

CHAPTER TEN

MENTAL ENGAGEMENT: KEEPING THE MIND SHARP

Talking about the above, our search light shall be upon the link between mental activity and cognitive health in aging, outlining brain-training exercises, lifelong learning, and fostering social connections.

Maintaining mental engagement and cognitive activity is crucial for promoting cognitive health and preserving mental sharpness as individuals age. There is a strong link between mental activity, brain health, and cognitive function. Here's an exploration of the importance of mental engagement in aging, along with strategies such as brain-training exercises, lifelong learning, and fostering social connections:

Neuroplasticity and Cognitive Health:

Neuroplasticity refers to the brain's ability to reorganize and form new neural connections throughout life.

Engaging in mentally stimulating activities can enhance neuroplasticity, supporting cognitive function and potentially delaying cognitive decline.

Brain-Training Exercises:

Cognitive Training Apps: Various apps and online programs offer games and exercises designed to challenge memory, attention, and problem-solving skills.

Puzzles and Games: Activities like crossword puzzles, Sudoku, and chess can stimulate the brain and provide a enjoyable way to engage mentally.

Memory Techniques: Practicing mnemonic devices and memory techniques can help enhance memory and cognitive skills.

Lifelong Learning:

Formal Education: Pursuing formal education or taking courses later in life can provide mental stimulation and promote continuous learning.

Reading: Regular reading, whether books, articles, or newspapers, exposes the brain to new information and ideas.

Learning a New Skill or Hobby: Acquiring a new skill, whether it's playing a musical instrument, learning a language, or taking up a craft, provides mental challenges that contribute to cognitive health.

Social Connections and Cognitive Health:

Social Engagement: Maintaining strong social connections has been linked to better cognitive health. Engaging in social activities, group events, and conversations stimulates the brain.

Volunteering: Participating in volunteer activities not only fosters social connections but also provides a sense of purpose and mental stimulation.

Joining Clubs or Groups: Being part of clubs, discussion groups, or community organizations encourages ongoing social interaction and mental engagement.

Physical Activity and Cognitive Function:

Regular exercise has been shown to have positive effects on cognitive function. It improves blood flow to the brain, promotes neurogenesis (the formation of new neurons), and supports overall brain health.

Mindfulness and Meditation:

Practices like mindfulness meditation can enhance cognitive function by promoting attention, focus, and emotional regulation.

Balanced Diet and Brain Health:

Nutrient-rich foods, particularly those rich in antioxidants and omega-3 fatty acids, support brain health and cognitive function.

Adequate Sleep:

Quality sleep is essential for memory consolidation and cognitive performance. Prioritizing good sleep hygiene contributes to mental sharpness.

Regular Health Check-ups:

Monitoring and managing overall health, including conditions such as hypertension and diabetes, can contribute to cognitive health.

Stress Management:

Chronic stress negatively impacts cognitive function. Effective stress management techniques, such as mindfulness and relaxation exercises, contribute to cognitive well-being.

Adapting to Age-Related Changes:

Accepting and adapting to age-related cognitive changes, while still engaging in mentally stimulating activities, helps individuals maintain a positive and resilient mindset.

By incorporating these strategies into daily life, individuals can foster mental engagement, promote cognitive health, and contribute to maintaining mental sharpness as they age. Staying curious, being socially active, and challenging the brain with diverse activities are essential components of a holistic approach to mental well-being throughout the aging process.

CHAPTER ELEVEN

EMERGING TECHNOLOGIES: THE LONGEVITY TOOLBOX

Emerging technologies in biotechnology, gene editing, and personalized medicine are at the forefront of scientific research, offering promising avenues for understanding and potentially positively impacting aging and extending lifespan. While these areas of study are dynamic and ongoing, several developments show potential in the quest for healthy aging and increased longevity:

Senolytics and Senescence-Associated Therapies:

Senolytics are drugs designed to target and eliminate senescent cells, which accumulate with age and contribute to inflammation and tissue dysfunction.

Emerging therapies aim to develop drugs that can selectively remove these senescent cells, potentially promoting healthier aging.

Telomere Extension and Telomerase Activation:

Telomeres, protective caps at the ends of chromosomes, naturally shorten with each cell division. Telomerase is an enzyme that can elongate telomeres.

Research is exploring ways to activate telomerase to maintain or lengthen telomeres, potentially slowing down cellular aging and promoting longevity.

Gene Editing Technologies (CRISPR-Cas9):

CRISPR-Cas9 is a revolutionary gene-editing tool that enables precise modification of genes within an organism.

Researchers are exploring the potential to edit genes associated with aging, addressing genetic factors that contribute to age-related diseases and promoting healthier aging

Epigenetic Therapies:

Epigenetic modifications play a role in gene expression and aging. Emerging therapies aim to modify or reverse these epigenetic changes to rejuvenate cells and tissues.

Epigenetic editing technologies are being explored for their potential to reset cellular aging clocks.

Mitochondrial Therapies:

Mitochondria, the cellular powerhouses, play a role in aging and age-related diseases. Therapies are being developed to enhance mitochondrial function and mitigate the impact of mitochondrial dysfunction.

Strategies include targeting mitochondrial DNA, improving mitochondrial quality control, and enhancing overall mitochondrial health.

Microbiome Interventions:

The gut microbiome influences various aspects of health, including metabolism and immune function. Interventions such as microbiome modulation and fecal microbiota transplantation are being explored for their potential impact on aging and age-related diseases.

Personalized Medicine and Biomarker Identification:

Advances in genomics, proteomics, and other omics technologies contribute to the development of personalized medicine.

Biomarkers associated with aging and age-related diseases are being identified, allowing for early detection, personalized interventions, and monitoring of individual health trajectories.

AI and Machine Learning in Aging Research:

Artificial intelligence and machine learning algorithms are being used to analyze large datasets, identify patterns, and predict disease risk.

These technologies aid in understanding the complex interactions involved in aging and can contribute to personalized treatment approaches.

NAD+ Supplementation:

NAD+ (nicotinamide adenine dinucleotide) is a coenzyme involved in cellular energy production. NAD+ levels decline with age.

NAD+ supplementation is being explored as a potential intervention to enhance cellular function and slow down the aging process.

Therapies Targeting Aging Pathways:

Research is focused on identifying and targeting specific molecular pathways associated with aging, such as mTOR, sirtuins, and AMPK, with the goal of developing interventions that can slow down or reverse the aging process.

While these emerging technologies show promise, it's important to note that the field of aging research is complex, and ethical considerations must be taken into account. Additionally, the translation of laboratory findings into safe and effective clinical applications requires rigorous testing and validation. As the science evolves, ongoing research and collaboration among scientists, clinicians, and ethical experts are crucial for ensuring responsible and beneficial applications of these technologies in the context of aging and longevity.

CHAPTER TWELVE

THE ETHICS OF LONGEVITY

Living Longer, Living Better: Raise ethical considerations surrounding longevity research and interventions, exploring issues of resource allocation, equity, and potential societal implications.

As longevity research advances and the possibility of interventions to extend human life becomes more plausible, ethical considerations become increasingly important. Addressing these ethical concerns is crucial to ensuring that longevity-related developments benefit society as a whole. Here are some key ethical considerations surrounding longevity research and interventions:

Resource Allocation and Equity:

Access to Longevity Interventions: As longevity interventions become available, questions arise about equitable access. Ensuring that these interventions are accessible to diverse socioeconomic groups and not disproportionately benefiting the privileged is a critical ethical concern.

Allocation of Healthcare Resources: Longevity interventions may compete with other essential healthcare needs. Ethical decision-making involves balancing resources to address pressing health issues and promote overall well-being.

Societal Impact:

Population Aging: Longevity interventions could contribute to an aging population, potentially affecting social structures, workforce dynamics, and pension systems. Ethical considerations include addressing the societal implications of an increasingly elderly population.

Intergenerational Equity: Balancing the interests of different generations is important. Ethical frameworks need to account for the potential impact of longevity interventions on future generations, considering issues such as environmental sustainability and resource distribution.

Health Inequality and Disparities:

Addressing Health Disparities: Longevity interventions should aim to address existing health disparities rather than exacerbating them. Ethical research and interventions should prioritize health equity and consider the needs of marginalized communities.

Avoiding Enhancement Divide: Ensuring that longevity interventions are not exclusively available to a privileged few prevents the creation of an "enhancement divide" where only certain segments of the population have access to life-extending technologies.

Informed Consent and Autonomy:

Transparent Communication: Ethical longevity research requires transparent communication about potential risks, uncertainties, and benefits. Individuals should be fully informed about the implications of participating in studies or undergoing interventions.

Respecting Autonomy: Longevity interventions should respect individual autonomy. People should have the right to make informed decisions about their health, including whether to pursue life-extending interventions.

Definition of a Good Life:

Cultural and Personal Values: The definition of a "good life" varies among individuals and cultures. Ethical considerations include respecting diverse values and allowing individuals to define what a meaningful and fulfilling life means to them.

Unintended Consequences and Risks:

Unintended Societal Consequences: Ethical research must consider potential unintended consequences, such as increased social inequality or unforeseen impacts on family structures.

Unknown Long-Term Risks: Longevity interventions may have unknown long-term risks. Ethical research requires thorough investigation of potential harms and mitigation strategies.

Global Considerations:

Global Access to Benefits: Ethical considerations extend globally, with the need to ensure that the benefits of longevity interventions are accessible to people around the world.

Avoiding Global Inequities: Efforts should be made to avoid creating global disparities where only certain regions or populations have access to the benefits of longevity research.

Regulatory Oversight:

Ethical Research Standards: Establishing and adhering to rigorous ethical standards in research and development, including regulatory oversight, helps safeguard against potential harms and ensures the responsible progression of longevity interventions.

Balancing the pursuit of longer, healthier lives with ethical considerations is essential to create a future where longevity interventions contribute to the well-being of individuals and society as a whole. Open and inclusive discussions involving researchers, policymakers, ethicists, and the public can help shape ethical frameworks that guide the responsible development and deployment of longevity-related interventions.

CHAPTER THIRTEEN

RETHINKING AGING,A PARADIGM SHIFT

Advocate for a cultural shift in perceptions of aging, promoting active, engaged, and meaningful elderhood as a valuable stage of life.

Promoting a cultural shift in perceptions of aging is essential to foster a society that values and supports active, engaged, and meaningful elderhood. This paradigm shift challenges ageist stereotypes and encourages a more positive and inclusive view of aging as a valuable stage of life. Here are key elements to advocate for a cultural shift in perceptions of aging:

Positive Aging Narratives:

Encourage the creation and dissemination of positive aging narratives in media, literature, and other forms of storytelling.

Highlight stories of individuals who lead fulfilling lives, contribute to their communities, and pursue new opportunities in later years.

Challenging Ageism:

Raise awareness about ageism and challenge stereotypes that perpetuate negative views of aging.

Advocate for policies and practices that combat age discrimination in the workplace, healthcare, and other societal domains.

Embracing Diversity in Aging:

Celebrate the diversity of experiences within the older population, recognizing that aging is not a monolithic experience.

Highlight the contributions of older adults from various cultural, ethnic, and socioeconomic backgrounds.

Promoting Intergenerational Connections:

Encourage intergenerational interactions and collaborations to foster understanding, mutual respect, and the exchange of knowledge between different age groups.

Create opportunities for shared experiences that bridge generational gaps and build connections.

Valuing Wisdom and Experience:

Emphasize the value of the wisdom, experience, and accumulated knowledge that older adults bring to their communities.

Recognize and utilize the expertise of older individuals in mentoring, teaching, and advising roles.

Redefining Success and Productivity:

Challenge narrow definitions of success and productivity that focus solely on professional achievements or economic contributions.

Acknowledge and celebrate contributions to family, community, and personal growth as meaningful markers of success in later life.

Supporting Lifelong Learning:

Promote a culture of lifelong learning, emphasizing the importance of acquiring new skills, pursuing interests, and engaging in intellectual pursuits at every stage of life.

Encourage educational institutions and community organizations to provide accessible learning opportunities for older adults.

Active Aging and Well-being:

Emphasize the importance of staying physically active, maintaining mental well-being, and adopting healthy lifestyle habits throughout the aging process.

Showcase examples of older individuals leading active and fulfilling lives through sports, hobbies, and recreational activities.

Cultivating Purpose and Meaning:

Advocate for the recognition of the need for purpose and meaning in later life.

Support programs and initiatives that help older individuals find and pursue activities that bring fulfillment and a sense of purpose.

Age-Friendly Environments:

Advocate for the creation of age-friendly communities that accommodate the needs and preferences of older residents.

Encourage urban planning and design that facilitates accessibility, social engagement, and inclusion for people of all ages.

Policy and Legislative Support:

Work towards the development and implementation of policies that promote the rights and well-being of older adults, including healthcare access, social services, and employment opportunities.

Advocate for age-friendly policies that address the diverse needs of an aging population.

By actively promoting these principles and challenging negative stereotypes, society can shift towards a more inclusive and appreciative perspective on aging. Embracing the richness of elderhood as a valuable stage of life contributes to building a culture that values and supports individuals across the entire lifespan.

CHAPTER FOURTEEN

INDIVIDUAL ACTION, COLLECTIVE IMPACT

Empowering individuals to take personal responsibility for their health and longevity is a crucial step toward fostering a culture of proactive aging. However, individual actions alone may not be sufficient; collective impact through public policy changes and scientific research advancements is equally essential for creating a society that supports healthy aging. Here's how readers can take individual action while advocating for broader changes:

Individual Action:

Healthy Lifestyle Choices:

Adopt a balanced and nutritious diet, engaging in regular physical activity, and maintaining a healthy weight contribute to overall well-being.

Avoid harmful habits such as smoking and excessive alcohol consumption.

Regular Health Check-ups:

Schedule regular health check-ups to monitor and manage health conditions.

Be proactive in addressing health concerns and seeking preventive care.

Mental and Emotional Well-being:

Prioritize mental health by managing stress, practicing mindfulness, and seeking support when needed.

Engage in activities that promote emotional well-being, such as hobbies, social interactions, and relaxation techniques.

Lifelong Learning:

Cultivate a mindset of continuous learning and intellectual curiosity.

Explore new skills, hobbies, and educational opportunities throughout life.

Social Connections:

Foster strong social connections by staying engaged with friends, family, and community.

Actively participate in social activities and contribute to building a supportive network.

Purpose and Meaning:

Identify and pursue activities that provide a sense of purpose and meaning.

Volunteer, mentor, or engage in projects that align with personal values and contribute to the well-being of others.

Sleep Hygiene:

Prioritize good sleep hygiene by establishing consistent sleep patterns and creating a conducive sleep environment.

Advocacy and Community Engagement:

Advocate for age-friendly policies and initiatives in local communities.

Engage in community organizations or join advocacy groups focused on health and aging issues.

Collective Impact:

Supporting Scientific Research:

Stay informed about ongoing scientific research related to aging and longevity.

Advocate for increased funding and support for research initiatives addressing age-related diseases and interventions.

Political Advocacy:

Stay informed about relevant policy issues related to healthcare, aging, and public health.

Advocate for policies that support healthy aging, access to healthcare, and research advancements.

Community Building:

Participate in or support community initiatives that promote healthy aging, such as senior centers, wellness programs, and community gardens.

Collaborate with local organizations to create age-friendly environments.

Public Health Campaigns:

Support and participate in public health campaigns that raise awareness about the importance of healthy aging, preventive care, and mental well-being.

Education and Outreach:

Share information and resources about healthy aging with friends, family, and community members.

Engage in educational outreach to dispel myths and stereotypes about aging.

Interdisciplinary Collaboration:

Advocate for interdisciplinary collaboration among healthcare professionals, researchers, policymakers, and community organizations to address holistic approaches to healthy aging.

Technology and Innovation:

Support the development and implementation of technological solutions that enhance healthcare accessibility, monitor health metrics, and improve overall well-being for older adults.

By combining personal responsibility with advocacy for broader societal changes, individuals can contribute to creating a supportive environment for healthy aging. Engaging in collective efforts amplifies the impact, fostering a society that values, promotes, and supports the well-being and longevity of all its members.

CHAPTER FIFTEEN

LIVING WITH PURPOSE: EMBRACING THE AGING JOURNEY

Conclude with a message of hope and optimism, offering practical guidance on finding meaning and purpose in every stage of life, while embracing the inevitable process of aging with grace and acceptance.

Embracing the aging journey is a transformative process that can be filled with purpose, meaning, and a profound sense of fulfillment. As we navigate the inevitable changes that come with aging, it's essential to approach this journey with hope, optimism, and a commitment to living with purpose. Here are some practical guidance and words of encouragement:

Cultivate a Positive Mindset:

Embrace a positive attitude towards aging. Recognize the wisdom, experience, and resilience that come with the passing years.

Focus on the opportunities for growth, learning, and joy that each stage of life brings.

Define Your Own Meaning and Purpose:

Reflect on your values, passions, and interests. What brings you joy and a sense of fulfillment?

Define your own meaning and purpose, and allow them to guide your choices and actions.

Continuous Learning and Curiosity:

Embrace a mindset of lifelong learning. Seek out new experiences, acquire new skills, and stay curious about the world around you.

Each day offers an opportunity for discovery and personal growth.

Connection and Community:

Nurture meaningful connections with friends, family, and community. Social engagement is a cornerstone of a purposeful life.

Share your experiences, wisdom, and stories with others, and be open to learning from their journeys.

Contribution and Service:

Find ways to contribute to the well-being of others. Engage in acts of kindness, volunteer, and share your time and skills with your community.

The sense of purpose that comes from making a positive impact is a powerful source of fulfillment.

Adaptability and Resilience:

Embrace the inevitability of change and approach it with adaptability and resilience.

Each life stage brings its own challenges, but also opportunities for growth and new beginnings.

Self-Care and Well-Being:

Prioritize self-care, including physical, mental, and emotional well-being. Take time for activities that bring you joy and relaxation.

Cultivate a healthy lifestyle that supports your overall health and vitality.

Mindfulness and Presence:

Practice mindfulness and be present in each moment. Appreciate the beauty and richness of the present, rather than dwelling on the past or worrying about the future.

Mindfulness enhances our ability to savor life's experiences and find joy in the ordinary.

Celebrating Milestones:

Celebrate the milestones and achievements of your life. Each stage is an accomplishment that contributes to your unique and evolving narrative.

Reflect on the lessons learned, the relationships built, and the legacy you are creating.

Graceful Acceptance:

Embrace the inevitability of aging with grace and acceptance. Recognize that aging is a natural part of the human experience.

Cultivate self-compassion and be kind to yourself as you navigate the physical, emotional, and spiritual aspects of aging.

In embracing the aging journey with purpose, each day becomes an opportunity to savor the richness of life, contribute to the well-being of others, and find fulfillment in the present moment. Remember that age is not a limitation but a badge of honor, marking a life well-lived. As you navigate the path ahead, may you find joy, purpose, and a deep sense of contentment, embracing the full spectrum of the aging experience with open arms and a grateful heart.